SLIMDOWN SMOOTHIES FOR BEGINNERS

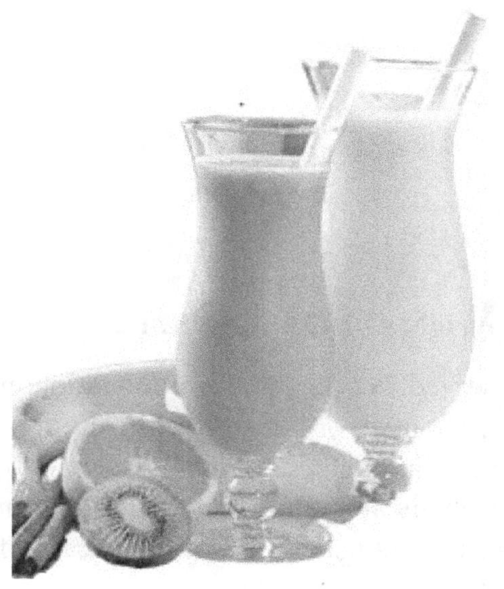

30 TESTED AND TRUSTED DELICIOUS RECIPES FOR WEIGHT LOSS

STEVE K. PARKINS

TABLE OF CONTENTS

INTRODUCTION

DELICIOUS SMOOTHES RECIPES FOR SLIMMING DOWN

INTRODUCTION

Jessica had always struggled with her weight. She had tried numerous diets and exercise routines, but nothing seemed to work. Frustrated and on the verge of giving up, she came across a book on slimdown smoothies. Intrigued by the concept, she decided to give it a try.

Jessica started incorporating slimdown smoothies into her daily routine. Each morning, she would whip up a delicious blend of fruits, vegetables, and other nutritious ingredients. Not only did these smoothies taste amazing, but they also kept her full and satisfied throughout the day.

Within just a few weeks, Jessica started to notice a change. Her clothes felt looser, and she had more energy than ever before. The numbers on the scale were steadily decreasing, and she couldn't believe the progress she was making.

Not only did the slimdown smoothies help Jessica shed the excess weight, but they also improved her overall well-being. Her skin glowed, her digestion improved, and she no longer experienced those mid-afternoon energy crashes. She felt revitalized from the inside out.

Inspired by her own transformation, Jessica began sharing her slimdown smoothie recipes with family and friends. They too started to see incredible results and couldn't thank her enough for introducing them to this simple yet effective weight loss solution.

Now, Jessica is on a mission to help others slim down and embrace a healthier lifestyle through the power of slimdown smoothies. Her story is a testament to the life-changing benefits of incorporating these nutrient-packed beverages into your daily routine.

If you're ready to shed those unwanted pounds and experience a new level of vitality, join Jessica on her journey. Grab a copy of the slimdown smoothies cookbook and start your own transformative story today. The power to slim down and live your best life is in your hands.

DELICIOUS SMOOTHES RECIPES FOR SLIMMING DOWN

1.Berry Blast

Ingredients

Filled 1 cup of mixed berries (Strawberry, blueberry, and raspberry)

one banana

spinach, 1 cup

Chia seeds, one tablespoon

almond milk, 1 cup

Ice cubes, if desired

Preparation

Blend the items together in a blender.

Blend till creamy and smooth.

If you wish, add ice cubes and mix one more.

Place in a glass and sip.

2.Green Goddess

Ingredients

spinach, 1 cup

12 an avocado

half a cucumber

a half-green apple

lemon juice from one

Coconut water, 1 cup

Preparation

Blend all the ingredients together in a blender to prepare.

Blend everything thoroughly and smoothly.

Pour cold liquid into a glass and serve.

3.Tropical Paradise

Ingredients

half a cup of chunky pineapple.

1/2 cup pieces of mango

half a banana

a tsp. of flaxseeds

Coconut water, 1 cup

Ice cubes, if desired

Preparation

To a blender, add all the ingredients.

Blend until smooth and creamy.

Ice cubes can be added if desired, then blend again.

Pour into a glass, then savor the tastes of the tropics.

4.Citrus Sunrise

Ingredients

1 orange, peeled

Peeled grapefruit, 1

Juiced lemon, half

1 teaspoon of honey

Coconut water, 1 cup

Ice cubes, if desired

Preparation

Blend the items together in a blender.

Blend everything thoroughly and smoothly.

If you wish, add ice cubes and mix one more.

Enjoy the zingy citrus notes after pouring into a glass.

5.Chocolate Delight

Ingredients

one banana, frozen

Cocoa powder, 2 teaspoons

1/4 cup almond butter

almond milk, 1 cup

1 teaspoon maple syrup or honey (optional for extra sweetness)

Preparation

In a blender, combine all the ingredients.

Blend until silky and creamy.

If desired, add honey or maple syrup after tasting.

Pour into a glass, then savor the delicious chocolate.

6. Mixed Berry Burst

Ingredients

Filled 1 cup of mixed berries (Strawberry, blueberry, and raspberry)

Greek yogurt, plain, in 1/2 cup

1/4 cup almond butter

almond milk, 1 cup

1 teaspoon of optionally sweetened agave nectar or honey

Preparation

To a blender, add all the ingredients.

Blend till creamy and smooth.

If desired, add honey or agave syrup after tasting.

Pour into a glass, then savor the berry taste explosion.

7.Creamy Green Apple

Ingredients

1 cored and chopped green apple

50 g of spinach

Slices of cucumber, 1/4 cup

12 cup almond milk without sugar

Greek yogurt, plain, in 1/2 cup

One tablespoon maple syrup or honey (optional for extra sweetness)

Preparation

Blend the items together in a blender.

Blend everything thoroughly and smoothly.

If desired, add honey or maple syrup after tasting.

Pour the cool green apple sweetness into a glass and enjoy.

8.Protein Powerhouse

Ingredients

1 scoop of protein powder in vanilla

Frozen banana, half

1/4 cup almond butter

1 cup of almond milk without sugar

a tsp. of flaxseeds

Preparation

To a blender, add all the ingredients.

Blend until it's smooth and well-combined.

Pour into a glass, and savor the energy boost that comes with the protein.

9.Peanut Butter Banana Bliss

Ingredients 1 banana, frozen

2/fourths cup peanut butter

almond milk, 1 cup

One tablespoon maple syrup or honey (optional for extra sweetness)

Ice cubes, if desired

Preparation

In a blender, combine all the ingredients.

Blend till creamy and smooth.

If you wish , add ice cubes and mix one more.

Pour into a glass, then enjoy the blissful combination of peanut butter and banana.

10.Minty Green Delight

Ingredients

A single cup of spinach

Fresh mint leaves, half a cup

Frozen banana, half

half a cucumber

a half-green apple

1 tablespoon of honey or agave syrup for sweetness

Coconut water, 1 cup

Preparation

Blend the items together in a blender.

Blend everything thoroughly and smoothly.

If desired, add honey or agave syrup after tasting.

Pour into a glass, and savor the flavor of the cooling mint.

11.Creamy Mango Banana

Ingredients

1 cup of chunks of frozen mango

one ripe banana

Greek yogurt, half a cup

coconut milk, 1 cup

1 tablespoon of honey or agave syrup for sweetness

Preparation

To a blender, add all the ingredients.

Blend till creamy and smooth.

If desired, add honey or agave syrup after tasting.

Pour the deliciousness of the tropics into a glass.

12.Blueberry Spinach Powerhouse

Ingredients

1 cup of blueberries, frozen

spinach, 1 cup

50 ml of almond milk

Greek yogurt, plain, in 1/2 cup

Chia seeds, one tablespoon

1 teaspoon maple syrup or honey (optional for extra sweetness)

Preparation

Blend the items together in a blender.

Blend everything thoroughly and smoothly.

If desired, add honey or maple syrup after tasting.

Pour the antioxidant-rich mixture into a glass and sip it.

13.Tropical Green Smoothie

Ingredients

1 cup of chunky pineapple

1/2 cup pieces of mango

spinach, 1 cup

a tsp. of flaxseeds

Coconut water, 1 cup

Preparation

To a blender, add all the ingredients.

Blend until it's smooth and well-combined.

Enjoy the tropical flavors after pouring into a glass.

14.Raspberry Coconut Refresher

Ingredients

1 cup of raspberries, frozen

50 ml of coconut milk

Greek yogurt, plain, in 1/2 cup

1 tablespoon of honey or agave syrup for sweetness

One-half teaspoon of vanilla extract

Preparation

Blend the items together in a blender.

Blend till creamy and smooth.

If desired, add honey or agave syrup after tasting.

Pour the cool raspberry treat into a glass, and sip it.

15.Smoothie made with pineapple and kale

Ingredients

One cup of finely chopped kale

12 cup of chunks of frozen pineapple

Frozen banana, half

1/4 cup almond butter

almond milk, 1 cup

1 teaspoon of optionally sweetened agave nectar or honey

Preparation

To a blender, add all the ingredients.

Blend everything thoroughly and smoothly.

If desired, add honey or agave syrup after tasting.

Fill a glass with the nutrient-rich green goodness after pouring.

16. Peachy Green Smoothie

Ingredients

1 pitted and sliced ripe peach

spinach, 1 cup

50 ml of almond milk

Greek yogurt, plain, in 1/2 cup

a tsp. of flaxseeds

Preparation

Blend the items together in a blender.

Blend till creamy and smooth.

Pour into a glass, then take a sip to enjoy the sweet and zingy flavors.

17.Banana Protein Shake with Chocolate

Ingredients

one banana, frozen

1 scoop of protein powder, chocolate

1/4 cup almond butter

almond milk, 1 cup

Ice cubes, if desired

Preparation

Blend all the ingredients together in a blender to prepare.

Blend until it's smooth and well-combined.

If you want, add ice cubes and mix one more.

Pour into a glass, then savor the delicious chocolate.

18.Berry Blast Smoothie

Half a cup of frozen mixed berries (strawberries, blueberries, and raspberries)

Greek yogurt, plain, in 1/2 cup

almond milk, 1 cup

1 tablespoon of honey or agave syrup for sweetness

Chia seeds, one tablespoon

Preparation

To a blender, add all the ingredients.

Blend till creamy and smooth.

If desired, add honey or agave syrup after tasting.

Pour into a glass, then savor the berry taste explosion.

19.Green Smoothie for Detoxification

Ingredients

A single cup of spinach

1 tablespoon freshly grated ginger,

 1/2 cucumber

1/2 green apple

1/2 lemon, juiced, and 1 cup coconut water

Preparation

Blend all the ingredients together in a blender to prepare.

Blend everything thoroughly and smoothly.

Pour the mixture into a glass, then use it to detoxify your body.

20.Lime Watermelon Cooler

Ingredients

2 cups of watermelon cubes

1 lime's juice

1 tablespoon of mint leaves, fresh

Coconut water, 1 cup

Ice cubes, if desired

Preparation

To a blender, add all the ingredients.

Blend until well-combined and smooth.

If you want, add ice cubes and mix one more.

Pour some watermelon and lime juice into a glass, then drink up.

21. Green goddess Smoothie

Ingredients

spinach, 1 cup

12 an avocado

sliced cucumbers, half

half a banana

1 tablespoon of lime juice, fresh

almond milk, 1 cup

Preparation

Blend all the ingredients together in a blender to prepare.

Blend until it's smooth and well-combined.

Enjoy the hydrating and nutrient-rich green smoothie after pouring into a glass.

22.Orange Carrots Glow

Ingredients

1 large orange peeled and segmented

1 medium carrot, cut after being peeled

Greek yogurt, half a cup

One tablespoon maple syrup or honey (optional for extra sweetness)

50 ml of almond milk

Preparation

Blend all the ingredients together in a blender to prepare.

Blend till creamy and smooth.

If desired, add honey or maple syrup after tasting.

Pour the colorful orange and carrot mixture into a glass and savor it.

23.Coconut Matcha Smoothie

Ingredients

1 cup coconut milk

1 tsp of matcha powder

Frozen banana, half

1 tablespoon of honey or agave syrup for sweetness

One-half teaspoon of vanilla extract

Preparation

Blend all the ingredients together in a blender to prepare.

Blend everything thoroughly and smoothly.

If desired, add honey or agave syrup after tasting.

Pour the creamy and antioxidant-rich matcha mixture into a glass and enjoy.

24. Pineapple Turmeric Refresher

Ingredients

1 cup frozen pineapple chunks

50 ml of coconut water

One-half teaspoon of turmeric powder

1/4 teaspoon ginger, grated

1/2 lemon juice

Preparation

Blend all the ingredients together in a blender to prepare.

Blend until well-combined and smooth.

Pour the exotic pineapple with a hint of turmeric into a glass and savor.

25. Cherry Almond Smoothie

Ingredients

1 cup frozen cherries

50 ml of almond milk

Greek yogurt, 1/4 cup

1/4 cup almond butter

1 tablespoon of honey or agave syrup for sweetness

Preparation

Blend all the ingredients together in a blender to prepare.

Blend until incorporated and creamy.

If desired, add honey or agave syrup after tasting.

Pour the delectable concoction of cherries and almonds into a glass and savor it.

26.Mango Ginger Zinger

Ingredients

1 cup of chunks of frozen mango.

half a cup of orange juice

1 tablespoon of ginger, grated

One-half teaspoon of turmeric powder

1/2 teaspoon of honey or agave syrup for sweetness

Preparation

Blend all the ingredients together in a blender to prepare.

Blend everything thoroughly until it's smooth.

If desired, add honey or agave syrup after tasting.

Enjoy the energizing mango and ginger combo in a glass after pouring.

27.Raspberry Beet Blast

Ingredients

1/2 cup frozen raspberries

chopped half of a tiny cooked beet

50 ml of coconut water

Greek yogurt, 1/4 cup

1 tablespoon of honey or agave syrup for sweetness

Preparation

Blend all the ingredients together in a blender to prepare.

Blend until it's smooth and well-combined.

If desired, add honey or agave syrup after tasting.

Pour the colourful, antioxidant-rich smoothie into a glass and savor it.

28.Kiwi Spinach Delight

Ingredients

2 kiwis, cut and peeled

spinach, 1 cup

Frozen banana, half

50 ml of almond milk

1 tablespoon of honey or agave syrup for sweetness

Preparation

Blend all the ingredients together in a blender to prepare.

Blend till creamy and smooth.

If desired, add honey or agave syrup after tasting.

Pour the kiwi and spinach mixture into a glass and enjoy.

29. *Blueberry Basil Boost*

Ingredients

Blueberries, half a cup, frozen

50 ml of almond milk

Greek yogurt, 1/4 cup

1 teaspoon of basil leaves, fresh

1 tablespoon of honey or agave syrup for sweetness

Preparation

Blend all the ingredients together in a blender to prepare.

Blend everything thoroughly and smoothly.

If desired, add honey or agave syrup after tasting.

Enjoy the antioxidant-rich blueberry and cooling basil combination in a glass.

30.*Avocado Green Tea Smoothie*

Ingredients

ripe avocado, half

1 cup freshly brewed and chilled green tea

50 ml of almond milk

1 tablespoon of honey or agave syrup for sweetness

1/2 lime juice

Preparation

Blend all the ingredients together in a blender to prepare.

Blend until it's smooth and well-combined.

If desired, add honey or agave syrup after tasting.

Pour the creamy and nourishing avocado green tea blend into a glass and enjoy.

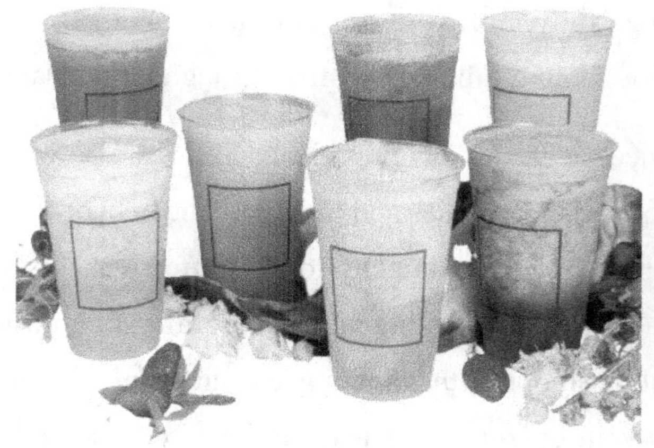

CONCLUSION

In conclusion, the Slimdown Smoothies cookbook is your ultimate guide to achieving your weight loss goals and embracing a healthier lifestyle. Packed with 30 delicious and nutritious recipes, this book offers a simple and effective solution to slimming down and feeling your best.

With the power of carefully selected ingredients, these slimdown smoothies provide your body with the essential nutrients it needs while supporting weight loss. Each recipe is thoughtfully crafted to not only taste delicious but also keep you feeling full and satisfied throughout the day.

The success stories of individuals like Jessica, who have transformed their bodies and lives with the help of slimdown smoothies, are a testament to the effectiveness of this approach. Imagine waking up each morning to a refreshing and filling smoothie that not only aids in weight loss but also boosts your energy levels and improves your overall well-being.

By incorporating slimdown smoothies into your daily routine, you'll embark on a journey towards a healthier, slimmer, and more vibrant you. Say goodbye to restrictive diets and hello to a sustainable, enjoyable way of nourishing your body.

So, whether you're just starting your weight loss journey or looking to break through a plateau, the Slimdown Smoothies cookbook is your go-to resource. It's time to take control of your health, revitalize your body, and achieve the slim, confident, and vibrant version of yourself that you've always desired.

Don't wait another day to start your transformation. Grab your copy of the Slimdown Smoothies cookbook now and let the journey to a healthier you begin. Cheers to a slim and vibrant life!

N.B IF YOU FIND DIFFICULTY IN PREPARING ANY RECIPE YOU CAN CONTACT ME FOR FREE CONSULTATION ON steveparkinshelpcentre@gmail.com